H
T

Method
For A Better Way
Of Life

How You Can Put Hidradenitis Suppurativa
Into **Remission**

By
Ignatz Rajher

Second Edition, 2019

Table of contents

Chapter 3: The three steps to put your Hidradenitis Suppurativa in remission 29

Prologue

What is Hidradenitis Suppurativa? Why did the medicine not yet manage to find the cause for it, even though the first diagnosis was already made in 1893? And even more important: How can it be that many of the people suffering from Hidradenitis Suppurative have been **successfully** treated while you have probably never heard of the information given in this book? How can it be that I wrote an article in 2012 to help many sick people, and yet I am one of the few authors in the world who are now writing about it again?

I had to realize that the life changing information in this book about Hidradenitis Suppurativa have not yet been spread wide enough, even after five years. Therefore, I decided to roll up my sleeves and to put a few lines on paper.

Please give me your trust and your attention for the next few pages and I will show you that you can also belong to these people who put their Hidradenitis Suppurativa in remission!

A new way of life awaits you!
As far as you decide yourself to take your life as well as your health into your own hand, to indulge my book without any prejudices and you decide to read a book concerning this subject for the last time – I will be able to help you!

Introduction

I am writing this book to show all people affected by Hidradenitis Suppurativa that there is a possibility to put their disease in remission (which means: the temporary or permanent alleviation of the symptoms of a disease). I am not speaking about a cure. I am sorry, we both **know** that there is no known/official cure up to this day. But I am also not speaking about the option to surgically remove the cysts and abscesses, just like the conventional medicine recommends you do. I am speaking about how YOU, with the help of this book, receive the opportunity to help yourself or your acquaintance to make the symptoms of the disease disappear **as long as you want**.

I am speaking about the following points:
- No abscesses anymore
- No cysts anymore
- No open wounds anymore
- No burning sensation anymore
- No feeling of shame anymore
- No suppressed anger anymore
- No suffering anymore!

I know I sound promising and at the same time you are afraid that I am just another one of these reckless merchants who are getting your hopes up just to get your money. Let me take this fear away from you by telling you the story of how I found the solution for this disease and what was the reason for me to write this book.

A long time ago

I was in a relationship with a woman once who I loved more than anything and for whom I'd have done anything. Since she was 18, she suffered from H.S (let's agree on this abbreviation for the rest of the book). Everything I wanted was that she was feeling well but living with this disease *can* turn a human into a different person. A person who, deep inside, is very sad, angry and possibly full of hate, sorrow and pain. She visited countless doctors and, apparently just like it is for you, nobody could help her. "There is no cure for that", "You're a case of one in a million" and even "Bad luck," are things she got from those doctors. All these words you would not expect from doctors. Which was shocking for me and made me angry. After years of watching without being able to do anything, I decided to end this suffering. The doctors and their statements, like "It's uncurable," made me enrage. Since I **knew** that something like "uncurable" doesn't exist, as long as a human is not missing something specific since birth or has been removed / severed in his life.

So, I set down at my computer and started looking for a solution for the problem. I didn't intend to close one eye before I had found a solution!

And three days later? I found a possible solution! I was absolutely amazed when I found it. Because I didn't have any clue at the start of my research, that this could be a way of "treatment". Everything I could find on the internet concerning this subject, was negative, depressing and did NOT help!

The only article that REALLY did do something, was the one I found on Tara Grant's blog (**Primagirl.com**), who suffered from HS herself for years. In two articles, she wrote how about how she managed to put her disease in remission for years now. Underneath, I found hundreds of comments from people who suffered from HS . People, who apparently managed to deal with their disease with her help as well. Jackpot, I thought!

After that, I printed the article to show it to my girlfriend back then. Full of anticipation to her reaction and the fact that I had found a treatment to an "uncurable" disease, I went to her to present this amazing news. Her reaction? More or less "What kind of bullshit is that? Who do you think you are, curing an uncurable disease? Get that shit out of my face".

Those were not exactly her words since it happened too long ago to remember them exactly. But that's exactly how it felt. Which motivated me to write down all the information in an article and to publish it on my (back then rather popular) blog www.true-words.eu in Germany. I thought to myself „If she doesn't want to believe me, then I might as well try to help others who are affected. After that, she just has to believe me!" 2-3 weeks after publishing my article "Hidradenitis Suppurativa: possible cure found" the article received SO many comments over weeks, in which affected people reported that already after a few days of using this method, the symptoms were gone, that she finally started to believe me. All's well that ends well?

This story doesn't have a happy end. She didn't seriously try to use my method and failed. While months after my publication of the article more and more comments of weeks, successful remission reports came in - I could not help *her*. The end of the story?

I felt as if I had failed entirely. I was able to help countless others and was overwhelmed with people thanking me, which, back then, didn't matter to me, to be honest, since I couldn't help the woman I loved. After a few months, I lost interest in my blog (which I ran for 5 years) and so the article disappeared from the net forever.

Why do I tell you this? Because I don't just not care anymore now and I want to help you and I also **can**. Five years ago, my article disappeared from the net and in the meantime, there was apparently no one in the German language area who considered it important enough to pass on this information. That's why I want to resume my original role and ask you with my story not to put your head in the sand like my girlfriend did and to surrender to your illness, but to take this information seriously and to actually **do** something with it. If you follow my method, you will get rid of the symptoms and a new feeling of life will arise in you again.

What's going to follow now is a more comprehensive version of my article. I am already looking forward to helping you in the next chapters, as long as you give me your confidence and really follow the steps. It will not be easy - but it will be worth it in the end!

Who the hell is this Tara Grant actually?

Tara Grant suffered from Hidradenitis Suppurativa for 25 years and experimented with different approaches for many years - until she actually found a solution. She rummaged through hundreds of clinical trials and found that HS is an autoimmune disease. Keeping a diet based on an autoimmune protocol in which she avoided certain foods for a certain period of time, she found her trigger-food after a period of time when the different kinds of food were gradually re-introduced into the diet: potatoes! By cutting out potatoes, she has managed to be in remission for more than two years. Even though this information has not yet arrived in mainstream school medicine, hundreds of commentaries on her blog, as well as numerous reviews of her book „**The Hidden Plague**", prove that she is right with her research, because many patients could – thanks to Tara- put their HS in remission. On her path of suffering, she visited over 40 doctors in four different countries and none of them seemed to be able to help her. All they told her was that she should continue to take her antibiotics, lose weight, they told her that she didn't wash herself frequently enough, she shouldn't wear tight clothing, try not to sweat so much and not wear Polyester.

No doctor has ever asked her whether this disease affects her interpersonal relationships or sex life. When she opened up and started to sob uncontrolled, she could tell how the doctors were tense and blocked her off.

They didn't want to talk. Either because they did not care or more likely because they could NOT HELP her. None of the doctors ever came up with the idea of transferring Tara to a psychologist or something like that, and to offer her spiritual help. People with HS can be depressed and even suicidal. Usually they are overweight (as they can move badly or exercise because of their pain), they miss a lot at work, can only move conditionally and have issues doing everyday tasks.

It took **15 years** for a doctor to make a diagnosis at all! Why? Because doctors were not sufficiently informed about this disease. Which is partly the fault of those affected. People with HS don't talk about their suffering, neither with their families nor friends. As Tara herself writes:

„We're suffering in silence and shame."
(The Hidden Plague, Pos. 288, Kindle Version)

After the failed doctor's visits and always the same answers, her HS didn't disappear, but only got weaker (if at all), she decided to somehow take her health into her own hands and began to look for a cure. She **did not** find any cure, but one way to put her HS in **remission**. According to her own data, she has been in remission for more than **two years** and no new bumps, cysts or abscesses have occurred. On the way, she also lost 35 kilos (from 107 kilogram to 72 kilogram).

Blog comments

I'll show you a few comments from the people who have read Tara's articles published in 2012 and thereby successfully put their HS in remission:

tonster (male) wrote on 28/03/2016 at 2:54 p.m.:

> *"For me, the cause is to 100% potatoes! I have been fighting with Hidradenitis Suppurativa for 20 years ... I was still in remission (while taking antibiotics) ... and suddenly symptoms broke out again .... I also realized what it was: potatoes! Already 12 hours later I could find some small spots on the body, which disappeared after a few days. The same happened to me a second time. And the third time I ate potato chips ... a few hours later - new bumps!"*

jojo5142 (female) wrote on 21/03/2017 at 10:49 a.m.:

> *"I just wanted to say I came across this article four years ago, and since then, I'm living free of Hidradenitis Suppurativa! I found out thanks to you that milk products are the triggers for me. Thanks to you, I could also help the daughter of a girlfriend who is only 16 and already suffers from HS I thank you so much for sharing your insights and history with us all! "*

Melanie (female) wrote on 25/04/2017 at 9:39 a.m.:

> *"Primagirl ... your article fascinated me when I happened to find it while I was looking for other things. I think, at the beginning, I didn't want to believe your article was true and only took a second look at it when the doctor diagnosed me with HS. I have been to many doctors for several years. Many of them had no idea what it. Some said "your body is just like that". Others gave me antibiotics, which did not help. And the last doctor gave me the diagnosis. " Hidradenitis Suppurativa".*

I HAVE NEVER HEARED OF THAT! When I tried to make sense of it on the net, I was quickly frustrated because there was no cure. Thus, years elapsed and the symptoms just did not disappear. Only after I came across your article, I thought to myself: "Wait a moment. POTATOES? This is one of the foods I have been keeping in my diet for years." I still did not want to believe your research and did not want them to work. However, I found it fascinating, so I decided not to eat potatoes that night. For a long time, I still ate no potatoes and the symptoms healed - no new bumps! Since I still refused to believe you, and thought that it was just a coincidence, I ate French fries two weeks ago, mashed potatoes and chips (I had a craving for it). And what happened then? SURPRISE. After many pain-free weeks, I am now again in a terrible situation due to new bumps and abscesses. I think now that denial and potatoes are no longer an option for me. I thank you for your blog ... "

Max Digger (male) wrote on 18.02.2014 around 7:25 p.m.:

"I just wanted to thank you for publishing this information. You have changed my life and I will always be grateful to you. I have already had two doctors and a big operation behind me. [There was a large part of the epidermal layer around the perineum (area between the anus and the external sexual organs] And no one in the medical area could tell me what the cause of this disease is, I had 10 post-surgical outbreaks at the operated area and took a bunch of antibiotics.

After I read your article, I ate Paleo and removed all the night shadow plants from my diet. Since then, I had no more outbreaks, no inflammations and lost 5 kilos. I also noticed how my Irritable Bowel Syndrome (IBS), which accompanied me for 15 years, disappeared at once. What a difference that makes up for my life! Blessed be you, keep going with the good work!"

I could go on like this all day and fill whole books with those comments, but I think you get my point. Other comments were also found under my article. Please, however, do not get the feeling that only nightshade plants work as triggers. There were also comments from people suffering from HS who addressed gluten, milk products and things like tobacco as a trigger. I hope that the comments motivate you to give me your trust for the time being. Let us first have a look at what Hidradenitis Suppurativa actually is.

Chapter 1:
What is Hidradenitis Suppurativa?

Acne Inversa (medical: Hidradenitis Suppurativa - abbreviation "HS") is a skin disorder in which the most sensitive areas of the body where skin to skin contact happens (under the armpits, genital area, between the legs, buttocks, underneath the breasts), painful abscesses, pus-filled cysts and hard knots are developed. Most people, on average, develop this disease at the age of 23 years. Women are affected 2 to 5 times more often than men.

The symptoms of bumps, abscesses, and cysts usually take months to heal. Sometimes these areas become infected and leave scars. These scars are not only on the skin, but also in the soul of the person concerned, since the disease has the following psychological effects. Sleep disorders, disgust, impairment of sex life, feelings of shame - especially in the social environment - are only some of the effects of this disease.

Stress, heat, hormonal changes, overweight, tight clothing and excess sweat may aggravate the symptoms, but **none of them causes** HS!

When the pus-filled cysts burst open, the symptoms spread to the skin regions in the immediate environment, but this does not mean that A.I. is contagious. It can't be transmitted from person to person. School medicine has no idea, what exactly the cause of HS is. All they have to offer are inefficient and sometimes temporary solutions.

Some of them are even very unhealthy for our bodies.

Hidradenitis Suppurativa, known since 1839

The first diagnosis to HS was made in the year 1839 by Alfred Velpeau. One might think that since then a lot of research has been carried out and the cause is about to be found out. Not even close. Do you know what happened in this area in the last 178 years? Nothing helpful. **NOTHING AT ALL**!

In 2000, Jan von der Werth published the article "The History of Hidradenitis Suppurativa" in the magazine "Dermatology in Practice" saying the following:

> *"Have we really failed to develop our knowledge of this disease, despite the powerful era of modern drugs and surgical techniques? I guess, in the eyes of many HS sufferers, the answer is "yes". May the one of you raise your hand, which is not discomfited when being confronted with A.I. patients. "*

In 1990, several detailed studies have shown that excess sweat becomes a problem when inflammation prevails but sweat is **not** the cause of the disease.

How many people are suffering from Hidradenitis Suppurativa?

There are allegedly about 70 million people affected worldwide. Of these alone, 225,000 to 3.1 million sufferers just in Germany. And 1 to 12 million in America.
Unfortunately, there are no exact numbers since most patients either don't get a proper diagnosis, don't go to the doctor because they are ashamed or can't be diagnosed, which makes them just estimates.
I advise every HS sufferer to go to the doctor to turn the estimates into real numbers.
If you enter the word "Hidradenitis Suppurativa" in Google Trends, you can see that the word has been googled in 42 regions of the world. For "Acne Inversa", there are even 58 regions. What does that mean? That the disease is a worldwide and not only a regional problem.

Chapter 2: Understanding Hidradenitis Suppurativa

Conventional medicine doesn't see the cause of illnesses in the diet of individual persons. They always pay attention only to the symptoms and the biological processes in the body, but never think about the fact that the diet could play a role and serve as a cause, too.

You've probably been to doctors several times. What did they tell you?

- "90% of the people affected by HS are smokers. Quit smoking. "
- "Most of the people affected by HS are overweight. Lose some weight. "
- "Don't wear tight clothing."
- "Avoid wet shaving."
- "I'll give you antibiotics." (Which did not help you, right?)
- "I'll give you a cream." (Which did not help you, right?)
- "The last option you will have is to take an operation into consideration" (The Internet is filled with reports that affected people who suffered from symptoms again after successful treatment - at the operated areas!)

That's all very helpful, isn't it? Why do they give you this useless information? Because the exact cause is still unknown today ... in **conventional medicine at least**!

I don't want to offend the school medicine. All I want is to reveal to you that there is a NOT OFFICALLY CONFIRMED but PROVED theory about what Hidradenitis Suppurativa actually is in truth. This theory is based on Tara Grant's article and her book "The Hidden Plague", which have been confirmed by numerous comments and reviews on her blog and her book. Just as through the comments in my article at the time. In order to understand what the true cause of Hidradenitis Suppurativa is, we first have to look at what's the deal with autoimmune diseases and how they function.

What is auto-immunity or why do you have to understand this process to conquer your Hidradenitis Suppurativa?

A properly functioning immune system is designed to protect us from harmful viruses and bacteria.
We all have molecules in our body that show the immune system that they are not a threat, and thus an intact immune system normally does not attack body-borne tissue either. However, if an autoimmune disease is present, the immune system can no longer distinguish between good and evil and starts attacking EVERYTHING randomly, causing damage to one's own body.

This process can cause autoimmune diseases such as:

- Alopecia areata (Circular hair loss)
- Antiphospholipid syndrome (APS)
- Asthma
- Atherosclerosis (arterial calcification)
- Autoimmune insufficiency, polyendocrine (subfunction of the parathyroid glands)
- Churg-Strauss syndrome (allergic granulomatous angiitis)
- Fibromyalgia
- Guillain-Barré syndrome (GBS - acute idiopathic polyradiculoneuritis)
- Hashimoto thyroiditis (autoimmune thyroiditis)
- Hepatitis, autoimmune (autoimmune hepatitis)
- Crohn's disease
- Multiple sclerosis
- Psoriasis
- Lupus
- Type I diabetes mellitus
- Vitiligo (Leucopathia acquisita)
- Celiac disease (gluten intolerance)

And many more. However, there are also diseases which are not officially regarded as autoimmune disorders, e.g. Schizophrenia, infertility, various forms of cancer and ultimately also Hidradenitis Suppurativa. What do they all have in common? In all these diseases the immune system is directed against the body (autoimmune reaction) and damages the internal walls of the intestinal tract. As a result, large quantities of unprocessed food enter the body. This is what is called a "permeable bowel" (Leaky Gut Syndrome). In doing so, the intestines such as proteins, pollutants, and bacteria from food enter the bloodstream. This should actually not be the case!

Many of these diseases are labeled as "old-age diseases" in medicine and are pre-treated as part of our normal life which is far from reality. These diseases have not existed a few decades ago and they are due to our unhealthy diet and our unhealthy lifestyle. Why do I think the school medicine will never take care of the treatment of such diseases (HS)? Because they do not consider the aspect of nutrition. As long as this circumstance doesn't change, there will be no official statements on the cause of HS and the knowledge you will take from this book will not penetrate the mainstream. The more familiar this book and its content becomes, the more likely is the chance that more and more people become aware of the cause of Hidradenitis Suppurativa.

What is the cause of leaky gut syndrome?

- Intake of antibiotics or cortisone
- Pathogens, e.g. Fungi and viruses
- Unbalanced diet (too much sugar, white carbohydrates, soft drinks)

It has been found that milk products, alcohol and cigarettes drastically help to develop a permeable bowel.

- Chemotherapy
- Heavy metals, e.g. Mercury through amalgam fillings in teeth

Connection between autoimmune diseases and HS

Let's talk about the connection between an autoimmune disease and Hidradenitis Suppurativa. For decades, scientists and doctors in school medicine have been picking up the wrong ideas, looking in the wrong places and drawing wrong conclusions. What exactly do they do? They are looking for a magic pill to cure the disease. But this is not the way Hidradenitis Suppurativa works! Scientists, doctors (who are ignored by the mainstream), recently published scientific studies and experts in the Primal / Paleo movement and came to a conclusion: A leaky gut (Leaky Gut Syndrome) is the main factor in the formation of autoimmune diseases.

People around the world have already managed to cure their autoimmune diseases, such as multiple sclerosis or rheumatoid arthritis, thereby gaining a new sense of life. They managed to do so alone, without the help of school medicine. They have cured their sufferings, which have been declared "permanent" by conventional medicine.

And without any medication or surgery. Exactly the same way you can also put your Hidradenitis Suppurativa in remission. When Tara Grant met Doctor Loren Cordain for the first time in 2011, she bombarded him with questions about her illness. He was the first doctor to refer to a possible connection between HS and a possible autoimmune disease. He saw countless clinical and anecdotal evidence that convinced him that Hidradenitis Suppurativa has auto-immunity as part of it.

What are the clues for that?

It could be proved that HS bumps have a high level of cytokines. Cytokines are proteins produced by the body's immune system that regulate the growth and differentiation of cells. A high level of this stuff in your blood triggers an immune reaction and your body begins to attack its own cells. Since this substance can be found in the bumps, we would here already have the first connection to an autoimmune disease.

Cordain also mentioned that the immune cells in the intestinal tract have become sensitive to proteins of certain foods. These immune cells start an attack every time these proteins (triggering foods) find a way into our body (through the permeable intestine), thus unintentionally destroying healthy cells. Since many people have already discovered that their symptoms are triggered by certain foods, this is another connection to an autoimmune disease.

Is there a definite curing method for a "permeable bowel"?

Unfortunately, there is no known, definite curing method. Even people who could treat their intestines have symptoms through certain foods and their proteins. However, as long as the human being avoids these foods, he does not suffer from the symptoms of his illness. So, when I speak of curing in this book, I am talking about a **remission**. Which is the case as long as the person concerned **does not eat** his trigger food!

The presumption that Hidradenitis Suppurativa is an autoimmune disease

It is thought that certain foods are the cause of the disease. As soon as you eat something that your body sees as a threat, your body begins to act with an autoimmune reaction and fights its own organism. In the case of Hidradenitis Suppurativa, abscesses and cysts occur. Nightshade plants are part of this group of triggers.

What are nightshade plants?

Nightshades are considered a trigger for inflammatory reactions in the body. People with a good immune system and healthy digestive tract are not affected. However, the substance "alkaloids" can destroy the cell membranes in some people and lead to overreaction of our immune system.

This increases the permeability of the intestine, which can lead to a permeable intestine. For the celiac disease (autoimmune disease), it has already been shown that gluten is the trigger and the phenomenon of the permeable intestine (Leaky Gut) can be blamed for this. Your goal will be to find out which foods trigger your Hidradenitis Suppurativa symptoms.

A list of the most common nightshades, known as triggers:

- Potatoes (all varieties other than sweet potatoes)
- Tomatoes
- Peppers (all types)
- Chillies
- Aubergines
- Goji berries
- All pepper varieties (except black pepper)
- Blueberries
- Andean berries
- Pear melons
- Lulo (Spanish Naranjilla)
- Tobacco / tobacco plant (Nicotine)

When buying food you will have to pay attention to the ingredients. In many processed products, for example, small amounts of peppers or tomatoes, as well as potatoes are used. If you buy something which says "spice mixture", you can assume that one of the nightshades will be contained in it. Learn carefully to read the labels of your food. If something should not be familiar to you - Google it.

Now you can say, of course. What? Tobacco? Does that mean I have to quit smoking? Most likely: "Yes". But don't start panicking now. Each person affected to HS reacts differently to the triggering nightshades. For one it's tomatoes, for the other one it's peppers, potatoes and so on. Sometimes others struggle with other known autoimmune substances, such as milk products. Sometimes it's the combination of several foods. In the next chapter you will learn the 3 steps that will let you find **YOUR PERSONAL** triggers.

If you do not achieve any success, think seriously about quitting smoking. Even if it is not a trigger for you personally, your skin will regenerate much faster. My advice to you for this project?
"Easyway to Stop Smoking" by Allen Carr

Summary:
How Hidradenitis Suppurativa works

To put it as simply as possible: The cause of acne Inversa is that it is an autoimmune disease. The known symptoms are caused by the fact that substances enter the blood circulation (because the intestine has become permeable) and are attacked by the immune system. In this attack, the immune system inadvertently damages healthy tissue because it fires wildly. Through the damage to the healthy body the well-known symptoms arise, which represent a mirror of the inner destruction and the body thus tries to give the humans a warning sign that something inside the body is not correct and is to be repaired.

If one makes the effort to look for the trigger food, which forces the immune system to randomly attack - the symptoms also disappear. So, let's get back to the 3 steps, which will put you in remission, as long as you **really use them**.

Chapter 3: The three steps to put your Hidradenitis Suppurativa in remission

Step 1: Elimination phase

Start by strictly eating food according to an autoimmune protocol. Eat for **at least 30 days** after this protocol. You will **most likely** notice a remission of your HS. Besides, you will feel incredibly good and even lose some weight-which is not our goal, but is just a nice by-product.

If a remission has not yet occurred, you have to take a closer look at your diet and see what else you can remove from your diet.

What does an autoimmune protocol look like?
There are different protocols (mostly Paleo-autoimmune protocols). However, for HS, I recommend you do without the following foods for at least 30 days:

- Nightshades (the most important renunciation of all!)
- Eggs
- Cereals (including rice and maize)
- Pseudo-cereals (amaranth, buckwheat, quinoa)
- Milk and milkproducts
- Nuts
- seeds (including coffee and cocoa)
- Non-steroidal anti-inflammatory drugs (contained in medicines such as aspirin and ibuprofen)
- alcohol (known for triggering the "Leaky-Gut" syndrome)

I know you're hating me right now just as I tell you to avoid most of your favorite foods. But keep in mind that it's only a phase until you find your triggers. If this task seems overwhelming to you at the beginning, then begin to sweep out the food which seems to be the most important trigger to people affected by HS.

Which are:

- Potatoes
- Tomatoes
- Paprika
- Chillies
- Aubergines
- Milk and milk products
- Gluten (in cereals)

If you can AT LEAST avoid these foods for the next 30 days, you could be among the majority of people who could uncover which foods work a trigger for themselves.

What could you eat in the meantime?

- High-quality meat would be recommended (beef, exclusively from grazing, etc.). But at the beginning, every meat that is not marinated or seasoned, which must be avoided, is fine.
- Offal and organics (including liver, heart, kidneys)
- Fish and seafood
- Vegetables of all kinds (as diverse and colorful as long as there are no nightshades!)
- High-quality grease (olive oil, avocado oil, coconut oil, fat fish, fat from pasturing)
- Fruits

I know the topic of nutrition can be very confusing and tiring. A change of diet is for most people a "pain in the ass". But I recommend you visit the website **thepaelodiet.com** to find out more about the Paleo diet.

Step 2: Reintroduce the food

As soon as 30 (even better 60) days have elapsed without new symptoms occurring, you will start gradually re-introducing individual foods into your diet.

Start with the second step when you can safely say that your symptoms are healing. Not sooner! If symptoms do not improve, take a closer look at your diet and see what else you can eliminate.

Keep in mind for the food you reintroduce: **ONE** after another! Each new food should be introduced **7 days** after the last one was. If you make the mistake of introducing two kinds of food within 7 days, and symptoms occur again, you will not be able to say with certainty which of the two is to blame. This means that you have to have patience and take your time for this process! Some people will experience symptoms after only 24 hours and one single intake, some only after days. This is the misleading thing about the disease. Therefore, you must follow these steps very carefully!

Eat the food 3 days in a row (first day a little, the second a little more and the third exaggerate - for breakfast, lunch and dinner) and wait for the following 4 days without eating it any further. See if something happened or not (so the 7 days come together). If there are no new symptoms, you can consider this food as "safe" after 7 days and incorporate it into your diet again. Afterwards, the search continues until you find a food on which your body responds with HS.

I would recommend to start in the following order:
- Potatoes (the most common cause among HS)
- Paprika (second most common trigger)
- Tomatoes (third most frequent trigger)
- Milk and milk products
- Gluten (in cereals)

If none of these foods is your trigger, go through the list of night shadow plants and the autoimmune protocol.

Most people whose trigger is a nightshades usually have symptoms with gluten and dairy products as well.

Do not trust your memory

It is of **great** importance to keep a food diary. Do not rely on your memory! Most people do not even know what they have eaten yesterday, how can you remember back what you ate in 3 or 4 days? No matter how well you think you can trust your memory. Leave it! Here are two options:

First:
Write an old-fashioned diary in which you write down WHEN and HOW MUCH you have eaten OF WHAT. And above all, how you feel in the morning after getting up, whether new symptoms have occurred and whether a healing process already takes place. Just as well, you could use a note app on your phone.

Example for an entry:
9:10 - 2 Eggs, 1 wholemeal bread, 1 tomato, cup of coffee

Or second:
Are you a friend of Smartphone Apps? Excellent! Search in Google Play Store for the free app "**MyFitnessPal**" and start using it. Personally, I prefer Option 2, because it is easier for me than to carry a book and pencil around with me.

Step 3: Successful remission phase

Once you've figured out what your "trigger food" is
DO NOT EAT IT ANYMORE!

It is so simple. If you don't eat the "triggers", you will not experience any symptoms. You can, however, experiment with it and see how many days in a row you have to eat the "trigger" to suffer symptoms. Some people will react very quickly to their triggers and some only after frequent / longer consumption. How many days in a row do you have to eat the food before new symptoms have occurred? Everybody will react differently. Get to know your body. And above all, as soon as you have clarity about your "trigger food"...

STOP! EATING! THEM!

As long as you stick to it, you will not find any new bumps, abscesses, or cysts, and a new life will begin for you. You have to realize one thing: After you have found your triggers, you should not consider your diet as a "diet", but put as much effort as possible into working out **your own** diet. What can you eat and what not?

Each HS affected will react differently and will be able to compile his own food plan for the rest of his life. So, do not make the mistake to look at it as some kind of sprint but more like a marathon. After all, you will need to avoid certain foods for the rest of your life to be symptom-free. Because, as already mentioned, this book **does not** offer healing, but only a way to get in remission. But this path will be free of pain, shame, disgust and depression. But with hope, new energy, a new way of life and a lot of joy for the rest of your life!

What you can do in the meantime against the abscesses

Coconut oil is known for its numerous positive effects on the skin. Its antibacterial and antimicrobial effect is due to the many amino acids, vitamins and trace elements.

> *"With whose help it is not only able to alleviate superficial suffering. Coconut oil is even able to heal degenerative diseases of the nervous system. "*

> *– Coconutoil.info*

So, I recommend you to put coconut oil on your abscesses to accelerate the healing process significantly. In order to ensure a high quality, it has to be Native, cold pressed oil.

Concluding words

The knowledge that Hidradenitis Suppurativa is an autoimmune disease is, unfortunately, very, very low. So, I wrote this short book about it. I know it will serve you well, if you follow the method.

I wish you a lot of perseverance and the greatest and fastest success in finding your trigger foods.

P.S.: I would like to know what you think about this book. Did you liked it? Do you hate it? Did it changed something deep down in you? Did it motivate you? Was it informative? Was it a waste of money, or the best money you have ever spent in your life?

Please take a few minutes and make sure to leave a review on amazon. I would appreciate your opinion a lot, because I read **every** new review that appears. And I am looking forward to read yours, too. No matter if you give it a good or bad review, **your opinion counts** - to *me*, and to *all* other future readers, that don't know if they should by this book or not. I know that you understand this. I would thank you for taking a few minutes out of your life to leave a review!

Imprint

Ignatz Rajher

Parlweg 4A

30419, Hannover

Germany

Email: ignatzrajherpublishing@gmx.de

Facebook Group

Facebook Group name: „Hidradenitis Suppurativa:The 3-Steps Method For A Better Way Of Life-Group"

Link:
https://www.facebook.com/groups/156702318259832/

If you want to connect with likeminded and share your successes or problems - feel free to join!

Password is: NOMOREHS

Made in the USA
Lexington, KY
05 August 2019